NATURAL REMEDIES TO REVERSE HAIR LOSS

UNLOCKING NATURE'S SECRETS - YOUR GUIDE TO RECLAIMING LUSCIOUS LOCKS WITH DIY RECIPES FOR HAIR GROWTH BLEND WITH POWERFUL AND CARRIER OILS.

GLORIA ACKLEY

TABLE OF CONTENT

INTRODUCTION

In the ever-evolving landscape of beauty and wellness, the quest for healthy hair stands as a timeless pursuit. However, for many people dealing with hair loss, gaining and maintaining beautiful locks can feel like an unreachable ambition. In response to this difficulty, there has been a renewed interest in natural therapies, which provide a holistic approach to hair loss treatment that prioritizes nourishment, balance, and wellness.

A variety of reasons can cause hair loss, including thinning strands, receding hairlines, and bald patches. Hair loss can be caused by a variety of factors, including genetic predispositions, hormone imbalances, stress, dietary inadequacies, and environmental aggressors. Recognizing the varied nature of the problem, natural therapies provide a comprehensive toolkit for combating hair loss from multiple angles, addressing both symptoms and underlying causes.

In this comprehensive guide, we embark on a journey through the realm of natural remedies to reverse hair loss. Our journey begins by delving into the complex interplay of lifestyle factors and hair health, shedding light on the profound impact of nutrition, stress management, and overall well-being on the vitality of our tresses. Understanding how our lifestyle choices can either promote or degrade the health of our hair lays the groundwork for accepting holistic remedies that address mind, body, and spirit.

As we navigate the complex network of hair loss reasons, we'll learn about the science behind natural therapies, including the medicinal capabilities of botanical extracts, essential oils, and time-honored techniques passed down through generations. From the relaxing benefits of herbal infusions to the invigorating effects of scalp massages and aromatherapy, each cure has the potential to revitalize the scalp, stimulate hair growth, and restore balance to the hair follicles.

Throughout our exploration, we'll emphasize the importance of consistency—a guiding principle that underpins the efficacy of natural remedies for hair loss reversal. While instant pleasure may elude us in the world of natural hair care, a consistent commitment to a holistic regimen provides noticeable effects over time. By incorporating natural therapies into our daily rituals with mindfulness and commitment, we create an atmosphere that promotes long-term hair health and vitality.

Beyond aesthetics, the path to cure hair loss with natural therapies is a significant act of self-care, affirming our innate connection to nature's rhythms and the knowledge of ancient healing traditions. It's an opportunity to retake control over our health, to cultivate a connection with our hair based on compassion and respect for its inherent beauty and strength.

So, whether you're dealing with the early stages of hair loss or looking to strengthen your locks for future issues, this book will serve as a beacon of knowledge and empowerment on your hair care path. By embracing the transformational power of natural treatments and building a lifestyle that values the subtle dance of body, mind, and spirit, you can achieve bright, thriving hair that represents the vibrant essence of your true self.

With each stride ahead, may you find inspiration, healing, and joy in the caring embrace of nature's remedies, and may your journey be guided by a firm belief in the ability of holistic wellness to illuminate the path to reversing hair loss and radiant vitality.

CHAPTER ONE

Understanding Hair Loss

Hair loss is a frequent worry that affects millions of people throughout the world, and it can be caused by a variety of circumstances. Understanding the various forms and reasons for hair loss is critical for successful management and eventual reversal. To begin, hair loss can present in a variety of ways, such as gradual thinning, patchy bald areas, or excessive shedding. These variances frequently imply separate underlying reasons, necessitating individualized treatment strategies. Second, a variety of causes can cause hair loss, including genetic predispositions, hormonal imbalances, lifestyle decisions, and environmental effects. For example, androgenetic alopecia, often known as male or female pattern baldness, is mostly inherited and affects both genders. Alopecia areata, for example, is caused by autoimmune responses that target hair follicles. Understanding these distinctions enables people to effectively address hair loss, whether by lifestyle changes, natural therapies, or medicinal interventions customized to their specific kind and cause of hair loss.

Hair loss, also known as alopecia, is a multidimensional disorder with diverse patterns, causes, and potential therapies. Understanding the various types of hair loss is critical for proper diagnosis and management. Let's take a comprehensive look at each type:

Androgenic alopecia

Androgenetic alopecia, often known as male or female pattern baldness, is the most common kind of hair loss among both men and women. It is mostly inherited, resulting from a mix of genetic predisposition and hormonal influences. In men, it usually starts with a receding hairline and thinning at the crown before proceeding to partial or total baldness. Women with androgenetic alopecia frequently exhibit generalized thinning of the hair on the crown while maintaining the hairline. The fundamental mechanism involves the hormone dihydrotestosterone (DHT), which shrinks hair follicles, resulting in shorter and finer hair growth cycles.

Alopecia Areata.

Alopecia areata is an autoimmune disorder that causes unexpected hair loss in isolated regions. It occurs when the body's immune system erroneously targets hair follicles, interfering with the regular hair development cycle. The specific etiology of alopecia areata is unknown; however genetic predisposition and environmental factors are thought to play a role. In some circumstances, the disorder can develop into alopecia totalis (complete scalp hair loss) or alopecia universalis (loss of all body hair). Stress, illness, or stressful events can worsen the disease, resulting in unpredictable hair loss patterns.

Telogen Effluvium.

Telogen effluvium is a transitory kind of hair loss characterized by excessive shedding of hair from the scalp. It happens when a large number of hair follicles reach the telogen (resting) phase of the hair development cycle early, resulting in excessive hair shedding. Physical or mental stress, childbirth, surgery, severe sickness, and abrupt weight loss are all common triggers. Telogen effluvium often begins two to four months following the triggering event, with visible hair thinning. Fortunately, the problem is treatable, and hair growth typically returns after the underlying cause is addressed.

Traction Alopecia

Traction alopecia is caused by long-term or repetitive tension on the hair follicles, which is frequently caused by tight hairstyles like ponytails, braids, or extensions. Repeated pulling causes damage and thinning of the hair shaft, resulting in hair loss, especially along the hairline or in areas of strain. Traction alopecia is common among people who routinely use tight hairstyling techniques or use heavy hairpieces. Early detection and prevention of hair-damaging activities are critical for preventing permanent hair loss.

Cicatricial alopecia (scarring alopecia)

Cicatricial alopecia, also known as scarring alopecia, is a condition in which inflammation destroys hair follicles and replaces them with scar tissue. This type of irreversible hair loss can be caused by a variety of underlying conditions, such as autoimmune illnesses, infections, or scalp trauma.

Unlike other types of hair loss, cicatricial alopecia causes permanent hair loss and scalp scarring. Treatment options are limited, with a primary focus on reducing inflammation and preventing scarring.

Anagen Effluvium.

Anagen effluvium occurs when the anagen (growth) phase of hair follicles is unexpectedly disrupted, resulting in rapid and severe hair loss. Chemotherapy, radiation therapy, and toxins are typical causes of anagen effluvium because they target rapidly dividing cells, such as hair follicles. Anagen effluvium, as opposed to telogen effluvium, actively develops hair rather than hair in the resting phase. While hair loss is frequently severe, it is usually transitory, and hair regrows after the causal agent is eliminated or terminated.

Other Types

Other less common causes of hair loss include trichotillomania (a hair-pulling condition), nutritional deficiencies (e.g., iron, zinc, biotin), and medication-induced hair loss (e.g., chemotherapy medicines, anticoagulants). These categories may have particular triggers and management strategies based on their underlying reasons.

Understanding the different types of hair loss is necessary for accurate diagnosis and therapy planning. While certain types of hair loss can be reversed with lifestyle changes, dietary adjustments, or medical treatments, others may necessitate long-term management techniques to slow progression and stimulate hair regrowth. Consulting with a healthcare expert or dermatologist is essential for tailored evaluation and guidance on the best treatment options for individual needs.

Causes of Hair Loss

Alopecia, often known as hair loss, can be caused by a variety of factors, including genetic predisposition, underlying health issues, and lifestyle choices. Understanding the many reasons is critical for proper diagnosis and therapy. This is a full overview:

Genetic predisposition (androgenetic alopecia)

One of the most common causes of hair loss is a genetic tendency, namely androgenetic alopecia, often known as male or female pattern baldness.

Inherited genes have an important role in determining vulnerability to hair loss, with patterns differing by gender and ethnicity.

Androgenetic alopecia is caused by the hormone dihydrotestosterone (DHT) miniaturizing hair follicles, resulting in increasingly finer and shorter hair growth cycles.

Hormonal Imbalances

Hormone fluctuations can cause hair loss, particularly in situations like polycystic ovarian syndrome (PCOS), thyroid disorders, and hormonal changes during pregnancy, childbirth, or menopause.

Hormonal imbalances can alter the hair development cycle, resulting in excessive shedding or thinning of hair.

Medical Conditions and Treatment

Hair loss can be caused by a variety of medical illnesses and therapies.

Alopecia areata (an autoimmune condition), lupus, and scalp infections can all cause hair loss, whether locally or widely.

Chemotherapy, radiation therapy, and some drugs (for example, anticoagulants, and antidepressants) can cause temporary or permanent hair loss by disrupting the hair development cycle.

Nutritional deficiencies

Inadequate consumption or absorption of vital nutrients can have an impact on hair health and lead to hair loss.

Iron, zinc, vitamin D, vitamin B12, and biotin are among the most common deficiencies linked to hair loss.

Poor dietary choices, restrictive diets, eating disorders, and malabsorption syndromes can all result in nutrient shortages and hair thinning or shedding.

Stress and Emotional Factors

Psychological stress, worry, and emotional trauma can cause hair loss via a variety of methods.

Stress-induced hair loss can take the form of telogen effluvium, which occurs when an increased number of hair follicles enter the resting phase prematurely, resulting in excessive shedding.

Chronic stress can also affect hormonal balance, worsen inflammatory diseases, and harm general hair health.

Lifestyle Factors

Certain lifestyle decisions and practices might cause hair loss.

Excessive or prolonged stress on hair follicles from tight hairstyles (traction alopecia), frequent use of heat styling equipment, or harsh chemical treatments can damage hair shafts and cause breakage or loss.

Smoking, heavy alcohol intake and poor sleep habits can all harm hair health and contribute to hair loss.

Environmental Factors

Pollution, ultraviolet (UV) radiation, and extreme climate conditions can all damage the hair cuticle, resulting in dryness, breakage, and loss.

Chemical exposure from hair dyes, bleaches, and styling treatments with harsh components can potentially cause hair damage and loss.

Ageing

As people age, their hair development cycles may shorten, resulting in decreased hair density and thinning.

Age-related hormonal changes, decreased scalp circulation, and reduced hair follicle function can all contribute to hair loss.

Hair loss can be caused by a variety of factors, including genetic predisposition, hormonal imbalances, medical problems, nutritional deficiencies, lifestyle choices, environmental effects, and aging. Identifying the underlying cause of hair loss is critical for developing focused treatment techniques that address the main cause while encouraging hair regrowth and restoration. Consulting with a healthcare professional or dermatologist can help with a thorough diagnosis and individualized treatment of hair loss based on individual needs and circumstances.

Other factors

Autoimmune disease.

Alopecia areata and lichen planopilaris are examples of autoimmune illnesses that cause the immune system to wrongly attack hair follicles, resulting in hair loss. In alopecia areata, the immune system targets the hair follicles, causing sudden hair loss in small, circular patches on the scalp. Lichen planopilaris is a kind of scarring alopecia in which inflammatory cells assault the hair follicles, causing permanent hair loss and scalp scars. These autoimmune disorders can have a significant impact on hair growth, necessitating medical intervention to reduce the immune response and possibly boost hair regrowth.

Scalp Conditions.

Scalp diseases such as seborrheic dermatitis, psoriasis, and fungal infections can all contribute to hair loss by inflaming, itching, and scaling the scalp. Seborrheic dermatitis, which is characterized by red, itchy, and flaky areas on the scalp, can weaken hair follicles and cause hair loss if not addressed. Similarly, psoriasis, a chronic inflammatory skin condition, can produce scaling on the scalp, disrupting the hair development cycle and leading to hair loss. Ringworm (tinea capitis) and other fungal infections can also cause hair loss by breaking down the hair shaft and damaging the follicle. Proper diagnosis and treatment of these scalp issues are critical for restoring scalp health and stimulating hair regrowth.

Medical treatments

Certain medical therapies, such as chemotherapy, radiation therapy, immunosuppressive drugs, and acne medications, might result in hair loss as a side effect. Chemotherapy and radiation therapy target rapidly dividing cells, such as hair follicles, causing temporary hair loss known as chemotherapy-induced alopecia. Similarly, immunosuppressive medicines used to treat autoimmune illnesses might alter the hair growth cycle, causing thinning or loss. Certain acne drugs, such isotretinoin (Accutane), can induce hair loss as a side effect. Hair loss caused by medical therapies is usually transitory, and hair regrows once the therapy is completed or terminated.

Physical trauma.

Physical trauma to the scalp, such as burns, traumas, or surgical operations, can cause hair follicle damage and loss in the affected areas. Burns, whether caused by heat, chemicals, or radiation, can irreversibly damage the skin and underlying hair follicles, resulting in scarring, alopecia, and permanent hair loss. Similarly, scalp traumas, such as lacerations or puncture wounds, can disrupt the hair growth cycle and prevent hair regeneration. Surgical procedures, such as hair transplants or scalp reduction surgery, can also result in temporary hair loss due to stress on the scalp tissues and follicles.

Trichotillomania

Trichotillomania is a psychological illness characterized by recurring, uncontrollable cravings to pull one's hair, resulting in visible hair loss and bald patches. Individuals with trichotillomania may feel tense or anxious before ripping out their hair, followed by a sensation of relief or fulfillment. Repetitive pulling can cause severe harm to hair follicles, resulting in breakage or thinning. Trichotillomania frequently necessitates psychiatric therapy, behavior modification strategies, and support groups to address the underlying triggers and behaviors linked with hair pulling.

Endocrine Disorders

Endocrine disorders such as Cushing's syndrome, adrenal insufficiency, and hormonal imbalances can impair the normal functioning of the endocrine system, resulting in hair loss. Cushing's syndrome, which is characterized by excessive cortisol production, can cause thinning of the scalp hair and profuse body hair growth in women. Adrenal insufficiency, commonly known as Addison's disease, causes exhaustion, weight loss, and hair thinning due to insufficient cortisol production by the adrenal glands. Hormonal abnormalities, such as variations in thyroid hormones (hypothyroidism or hyperthyroidism) or androgens (e.g., in polycystic ovarian syndrome), can also impair hair growth and cause hair loss. Proper care of these endocrine problems is critical for restoring hormonal balance and promoting hair growth.

Medicine Interactions

Certain drugs, when used together, might interact and worsen hair loss as a side effect. Combining drugs known to cause hair loss (e.g., antidepressants, beta-blockers, anticoagulants) may increase the risk of hair shedding or thinning. Furthermore, combinations between drugs and underlying medical disorders might lead to hair loss. It is critical to speak with a healthcare practitioner or pharmacist about potential prescription interactions and side effects, particularly their effect on hair health.

Thyroid disorders

Thyroid problems, such as hypothyroidism (underactive thyroid) and hyperthyroidism (overactive thyroid), can interfere with thyroid hormone synthesis, which is essential for controlling metabolism, growth, and development. Imbalanced thyroid hormone levels can disrupt the hair growth cycle, resulting in hair loss. Hypothyroidism can cause hair to become thin, dry, and brittle, but hyperthyroidism can cause hair loss due to faster hair growth cycles. Thyroid issues must be managed properly by medication, lifestyle changes, and regular monitoring to restore thyroid hormone levels and stimulate hair regrowth.

Anabolic Steroid Abuse

Abuse of anabolic steroids for performance improvement or bodybuilding can disturb hormonal balance and cause hair loss, especially in men. Anabolic steroids are synthetic versions of testosterone that have similar effects on the body, such as enhanced muscle mass and strength. However, long-term usage of anabolic steroids can restrict natural testosterone production, resulting in hormonal imbalances and associated adverse effects such as hair loss, acne, and gynecomastia. Hair loss caused by anabolic steroid addiction may be reversible after discontinuing the drugs, but hormonal balance must be restored before hair regrowth may occur.

These additional factors can cause or exacerbate hair loss in individuals, either alone or in combination with other causes. Identifying the underlying cause(s) of hair loss is critical for creating an effective treatment strategy that is specific to the individual's needs. It is suggested that you consult with a healthcare professional to properly evaluate and manage your hair loss.

CHAPTER TWO

Lifestyle Factors and Hair Health

Lifestyle variables, particularly nutrition and stress management, play an important role in achieving optimal hair health. A well-balanced diet high in key elements like vitamins, minerals, and proteins offers the foundation for healthy hair development and maintenance. In contrast, persistent stress and poor nutritional choices can disturb hormonal balance, affect scalp health, and contribute to hair loss. Understanding the effects of nutrition and stress management on hair health is critical for developing proactive measures for strong, vivid hair.

Nutrition and Diet

Nutrition and food are important foundations that influence not just general health but also the quality and appearance of your hair. A well-balanced diet rich in vitamins, minerals, proteins, and fats promotes healthy hair development, strength, and resistance. Here's a detailed look at how nutrition and food affect hair health:

Proteins

Hair is mostly formed of keratin, thus getting enough protein is essential for good hair growth and maintenance. Proteins are crucial building blocks for the growth and repair of hair follicles. Protein-rich foods include lean meats such as chicken and turkey, fish, eggs, dairy products, legumes, nuts, and seeds. Incorporating a range of protein sources into your diet ensures that you get all of the important amino acids necessary for good hair health.

Vitamins

Vitamin A: This vitamin is required for the formation of sebum, an oily substance that hydrates the scalp and promotes hair health. Vitamin A helps to promote the growth and development of hair follicles. Sweet potatoes, carrots, spinach, kale, and liver are excellent sources of vitamin A.

Vitamin C: As a powerful antioxidant, vitamin C aids in the development of collagen, a structural protein that strengthens the hair shaft. Adequate vitamin C intake promotes the strength and integrity of hair strands while guarding against oxidative stress. Citrus fruits, strawberries, bell peppers, kiwi, and broccoli are rich in **vitamin C.**

Vitamin E increases blood circulation to the scalp, which promotes nutrition delivery to the hair follicles. Vitamin E is also an antioxidant, which protects hair follicles from free radical damage. Nuts, seeds, avocados, spinach, and sunflower oil have high levels of vitamin E.

Vitamin D: Vitamin D is required to maintain healthy hair follicles and support the hair development cycle. According to research, vitamin D insufficiency may be connected with hair loss diseases such as alopecia areata and telogen effluvium. Sunlight exposure, fatty fish (such as salmon and mackerel), fortified dairy products, and vitamin D tablets can all help you maintain optimal vitamin D levels.

Vitamin B Complex: B vitamins perform a variety of roles in hair health, including energy metabolism, scalp health, and red blood cell synthesis, which transports oxygen and nutrients to the hair follicle. Biotin (vitamin B7) is essential for hair growth and is found in foods such as eggs, nuts, whole grains, and bananas. Other B vitamins, such as B12,

B6, and folate, promote healthy hair development and can be found in meat, chicken, fish, leafy greens, and legumes.

Minerals

Iron: Iron is required for the production of haemoglobin, a protein found in red blood cells that distributes oxygen throughout the body, including the hair follicles. Iron deficiency can cause anemia, which can result in hair loss. Consuming iron-rich foods such as lean meats, chicken, fish, beans, lentils, spinach, and fortified cereals will help you maintain proper iron levels and promote healthy hair development.

Zinc: Zinc is important in a variety of physiological activities, including DNA synthesis, cell division, and protein synthesis, all of which are required for healthy hair. Zinc deficiency has been linked to hair loss diseases like telogen effluvium and alopecia areata. Oysters, beef, pumpkin seeds, lentils, chickpeas, and fortified cereals are all good sources of zinc.

Selenium: Selenium is an important trace mineral having antioxidant characteristics that help preserve hair follicles from oxidative stress and damage. Selenium also aids in thyroid hormone metabolism, which affects hair growth and quality. Selenium is found in a variety of foods, including seafood, whole grains, eggs, and poultry, but it is particularly abundant in Brazil nuts.

Magnesium: Magnesium is involved in more than 300 enzymatic activities in the body, including those that control protein synthesis and cellular energy production. Adequate magnesium levels are required to maintain scalp health and promote hair development. Nuts, seeds, whole grains, leafy greens, legumes, and fortified foods are good sources of magnesium in the diet.

Essential fatty acids

Omega-3 and omega-6 fatty acids are necessary fats that help keep the scalp healthy, promote hair development, and prevent hair loss. These fatty acids nourish the scalp, control oil production, and maintain the hair's natural luster and flexibility. Incorporating healthy fats into your diet, such as fatty fish (e.g., salmon, mackerel), flaxseeds, chia seeds, walnuts, and avocados, can help ensure that you get enough essential fatty acids.

Hydration

Adequate hydration is critical for general health and well-being, including the condition of your hair and scalp. Water aids in the transfer of nutrients to the hair follicles while also flushing away toxins and waste particles that can impede hair development. Dehydration can cause dry, brittle hair, so drink plenty of water throughout the day to stay hydrated.

Antioxidants

Antioxidants are substances that serve to neutralize free radicals and protect cells, including hair follicles, from oxidative damage. Incorporating antioxidant-rich foods into your diet can promote healthy hair growth and protect the hair shaft and follicles. Colorful fruits and vegetables such as berries, citrus fruits, tomatoes, carrots, and leafy greens are rich in antioxidants.

Healthy Eating Habits

In addition to focusing on specific nutrients, proper dietary habits are critical for maintaining general health and hair development. Some important principles of good eating habits are:

Whenever possible, choose whole, minimally processed meals to increase nutrient intake while reducing consumption of added sugars, harmful fats, and artificial additives.

Balance your diet by eating a variety of food groups such as fruits, vegetables, whole grains, lean meats, and healthy fats to ensure you get a diverse range of nutrients.

Avoid crash diets and excessive calorie restriction, as they can deplete your body of key nutrients for hair health and cause temporary hair loss.

Limiting sugary, processed meals and beverages, as these can cause inflammation and have a bad influence on hair health.

Nutrition and food are crucial in maintaining optimal hair health and fostering healthy hair growth. By introducing nutrient-dense foods high in proteins, vitamins, minerals, and vital fatty acids into your diet and practicing healthy eating habits, you can nourish your hair from the inside out and keep it strong and vibrant. However, it is crucial to realize that, while diet is an important aspect of hair health, individual factors such as genetics, hormone imbalances, and medical disorders can all influence hair development and may necessitate further attention from healthcare specialists.

Stress Management

Stress management is not only important for general health, but it also helps to keep your hair healthy. Chronic stress can cause a range of physical and emotional health problems, including hair loss. Understanding stress, its effects on the body, and practicing appropriate stress management practices are critical to maintaining hair health. Here's an in-depth look at stress management and its effects on hair health.

Understanding Stress: The body's natural response to perceived threats or challenges. When confronted with a stressful circumstance, the body initiates the stress reaction, also known as the fight-or-flight response. This causes a series of physiological changes, including the release of stress hormones like cortisol and adrenaline, an elevated heart rate, and greater attentiveness. While acute stress can be useful in some instances, chronic stress, which lasts for an extended length of time, can hurt health.

The Effects of Stress on Hair

Chronic stress can impair the regular functioning of the hair development cycle, resulting in a variety of hair-related disorders.

Telogen Effluvium: Stress-induced hair loss occurs when a large number of hair follicles enter the resting phase (telogen) and then shed. This might lead to visible thinning and temporary hair loss.

Alopecia Areata is an autoimmune disorder characterized by unexpected, uneven hair loss that can be induced or exacerbated by stress.

Trichotillomania is a compulsive hair-pulling disorder that is commonly accompanied by tension or anxiety, resulting in visible hair loss and bald patches.

Chronic stress triggers the release of stress chemicals like cortisol and adrenaline, which can contribute to hair loss.

High amounts of cortisol, in particular, can interrupt the hair growth cycle and lead to hair loss by

Shortening the anagen (growth) phase of the hair cycle.

Inducing inflammation in the scalp, which can harm hair follicles and prevent development.

Suppressing hormones that promote hair development, such as insulin-like growth factor 1 (IGF-1).

Strategies for stress management

Effective stress management practices can assist in reducing the detrimental effects of stress on hair health.

Consider the following strategies:

Mindfulness and Relaxation Techniques: Deep breathing, meditation, yoga, and progressive muscle relaxation can all help you relax and reduce stress.

Regular Exercise: Physical activity has been found to relieve stress and increase mood by generating endorphins, which are the body's natural feel-good hormones. Almost every day of the week, aim for 30 minutes of moderate activity.

Healthy lifestyle habits: Prioritize self-care tasks like getting enough sleep, eating a healthy diet, staying hydrated, and minimizing your coffee and alcohol consumption.

Social Support: Seek help from friends, family, or a support group to share your feelings and experiences and acquire a new perspective on difficult situations.

Professional Help: If stress becomes unbearable or uncontrolled, consult a mental health professional, such as a therapist or counselor, who can offer coping skills and support.

Mind/Body Practices

Mind-body activities, such as mindfulness-based stress reduction (MBSR) and cognitive-behavioral therapy (CBT), can be especially effective in stress management. These approaches are aimed at increasing self-awareness, strengthening coping abilities, and addressing negative thought patterns connected with stress.

Prioritizing self-care.

Making self-care a priority is critical for managing stress and sustaining overall health. This includes establishing boundaries, practicing self-compassion, engaging in activities that offer joy and fulfillment, and getting professional assistance when necessary.

Long-term Stress Management

Developing good coping mechanisms and adopting stress management practices into your daily routine might help you become more resilient to stress over time. Remember that handling stress is a continuous process, and you must be patient and compassionate with yourself as you face life's problems.

Incorporating stress management practices into your routine can improve hair health. By lowering stress levels and encouraging relaxation, you can help reduce the detrimental effects of chronic stress on the hair growth cycle. Furthermore, prioritizing self-care and implementing healthy lifestyle choices can benefit your overall well-being, including the health and appearance of your hair.

A holistic approach to hair care.

Taking a holistic approach to hair care entails addressing not only external aspects like grooming and hair products, but also internal ones like diet, hydration, and stress reduction. By fueling your body and mind, you can promote healthy hair development and keep your hair vivid and robust.

Seeking professional advice.

If you continue to have considerable hair loss or other hair-related difficulties after using stress management measures, you should consult a healthcare expert or dermatologist. They can assess your hair's health, detect any underlying medical concerns, and suggest appropriate treatment alternatives.

Stress management is vital for preserving both physical and emotional wellness, as well as the health of your hair. Implementing appropriate stress management practices, prioritizing self-care, and getting help when necessary can help lessen the detrimental impact of stress on hair health and increase overall well-being. Remember that everyone reacts differently to stress, so pick tactics that work best for you and implement them into your daily routine

CHAPTER THREE

Natural Remedies to Reverse Hair Loss

Natural therapies for reversing hair loss are promising, with an emphasis on herbal medicines and vitamins, scalp care and massage techniques, and physical activity. Herbal medicines and supplements use botanical extracts and nutrients to promote hair growth and scalp health. Scalp care and massage techniques improve blood circulation, which promotes nutrition delivery to hair follicles and reduces stress-induced hair loss. Furthermore, exercise and physical activity boost general circulation, increasing oxygen and nutrient delivery to the scalp and promoting hair development. These natural therapies offer excellent treatments for hair loss and promote healthier, thicker hair.

Herbal Remedies and Supplements

Herbal medicines and supplements provide natural alternatives for stimulating hair growth and addressing the many conditions that contribute to hair loss. These alternatives include botanical extracts, critical nutrients, and traditional therapies to improve scalp health, strengthen hair follicles, and encourage thicker, fuller hair. Here's an in-depth look at typical herbal cures and supplements, along with tips on how to use them effectively:

Saw Palmetto

Benefits: Saw palmetto is thought to inhibit the enzyme 5-alpha-reductase, which transforms testosterone into dihydrotestosterone (DHT), a hormone linked to hair loss. Saw palmetto, which blocks DHT synthesis, may help minimize hair thinning and encourage hair growth.

Usage: Saw palmetto supplements come in a variety of forms, including capsules, pills, and liquid extracts. The suggested daily dosage is between 320 and 640 mg, divided into numerous doses. It is critical to follow the dosing directions on the product label or speak with a healthcare expert for individualized advice.

Ginseng

Benefits: Ginseng contains adaptogenic qualities that help the body adapt to stress, which is a significant cause of hair loss. Furthermore, ginseng may improve scalp circulation and stimulate hair follicles, resulting in increased hair growth and thickness.

Usage: Ginseng supplements are available in pill and tablet form, and can be consumed orally. The recommended dose varies according to the formulation and concentration of active ingredients. It is recommended that you follow the dosing directions on the product label or seek advice from a healthcare professional.

Rosemary Oil

Benefits: Rosemary oil has antibacterial, anti-inflammatory, and antioxidant properties that improve scalp health and hair development. It can increase scalp circulation, strengthen hair follicles, and minimize hair loss.

Usage: Dilute rosemary essential oil with carrier oil like jojoba or coconut oil to reduce inflammation. Apply the diluted oil mixture directly to the scalp and massage gently. Let it sit for at least 30 minutes before shampooing. To achieve the best outcomes, perform this process multiple times every week.

Biotin

Benefits: Biotin, commonly known as vitamin B7, is necessary for good hair, skin, and nails. It strengthens the hair shaft, prevents breaking, and promotes healthy hair development.

Usage: Biotin supplements are available in capsule and tablet form, and can be consumed orally. The suggested daily dosage ranges between 2.5 and 10 mg. It is critical to follow the dosing directions on the product label or speak with a healthcare expert for individualized advice.

Aloe Vera

Benefits: Aloe vera includes enzymes that stimulate hair growth, hydrate the scalp, and relieve inflammation. It promotes scalp health, balances pH levels, and improves the general quality of hair.

Usage: Apply pure aloe vera gel directly to the scalp and massage gently. Leave it on for 30-60 minutes before washing with lukewarm water. For the best results, repeat this treatment multiple times per week.

Peppermint Oil

Benefits: Peppermint oil has a cooling impact on the scalp, which can aid in circulation, reduce inflammation, and encourage hair development. It also has antibacterial properties, which can help prevent scalp infections.

Usage: To avoid skin sensitivity, dilute peppermint essential oil with a carrier oil, such as coconut or olive oil. Massage the diluted oil mixture into your scalp and let it sit for 15-20 minutes before completely rinsing. Avoid making direct contact with the eyes.

Fish Oil with Omega-3 Fatty Acids

Benefits: Fish oil contains omega-3 fatty acids, which have anti-inflammatory characteristics that benefit the scalp and hair follicles. They aid in minimizing scalp irritation, strengthen hair follicles, and encourage healthier, thicker hair growth.

Usage: Fish oil supplements with omega-3 fatty acids are available in tablet form. The suggested dose varies according to the concentration of omega-3s. It is recommended that you follow the dose directions on the product label or seek help from a healthcare expert.

Green Tea Extract

Benefits: Green tea extract includes antioxidants that preserve hair follicles and encourage hair development. It may also reduce the activity of enzymes that cause hair loss.

Usage: Green tea extract supplements are available in capsule and tablet form, and can be consumed orally. The recommended dosage varies with the concentration of active substances. It is critical to follow the dosing directions on the product label or speak with a healthcare expert for individualized advice.

Pumpkin Seed Oil

Benefits: Pumpkin seed oil includes phytosterols, vitamins, and minerals, which promote hair growth and may help prevent hair loss. It nourishes the scalp, strengthens hair follicles, and promotes overall hair health.

Usage: Pumpkin seed oil supplements are available in pill or soft gel form and can be consumed orally. The suggested daily dose ranges from 500 to 1000 mg. It is critical to follow the dosing directions on the product label or speak with a healthcare expert for individualized advice.

When using herbal therapies and supplements for hair health, remember the following:

Consult a healthcare practitioner before beginning any new herbal cure or supplement regimen, especially if you have underlying health concerns or are using drugs.

Follow the suggested dosage guidelines on the product label or as instructed by a healthcare provider.

It may take some time to see obvious results from using herbal medicines and supplements, so be patient and consistent.

Keep an eye out for any bad reactions or side effects, and stop using the product if you notice any.

Incorporate other healthy habits, such as a balanced diet, frequent exercise, and stress management strategies, to provide overall hair health support.

By including herbal treatments and supplements in your hair care regimen and adhering to these suggestions, you can encourage healthy hair growth and manage hair loss concerns naturally and holistically.

Scalp Care and Massage Techniques

Scalp care and massage practices are essential for fostering healthy hair development, keeping the scalp healthy, and preventing hair loss. By incorporating these techniques into your daily hair care routine, you may improve blood circulation, remove pollutants, and create an ideal environment for hair follicles to develop. Here's a full look at scalp care and massage techniques, including their advantages and how to efficiently include them into your hair care routine:

Benefits of Scalp Care and Massage

Scalp massage improves blood circulation to the scalp, supplying vital nutrients and oxygen to the hair follicles.

This increased circulation nourishes the follicles, promoting healthy hair growth.

Stress Reduction: Scalp massage promotes relaxation and relieves tension in the scalp muscles. Lower stress levels can help prevent hair loss caused by stress-induced hormonal abnormalities.

Exfoliation and Cleansing: Proper scalp care removes dead skin cells, excess oil, and product buildup, preventing clogged follicles and maintaining a clean, healthy scalp.

Scalp massage promotes the absorption of hair care products including oils, serums, and treatments, allowing them to reach deep into the scalp and hair follicles for optimal effectiveness.

Scalp Care Techniques.

Regular Cleansing: Use a gentle shampoo to keep your scalp clean and clear of pollutants. Choose a shampoo that is appropriate for your hair type and scalp health, and avoid harsh substances that might deplete the scalp's natural oils.

Exfoliation: Use a scalp scrub or exfoliating treatment once or twice a month to get rid of dead skin cells and product accumulation. Gently massage the exfoliant into your scalp in circular strokes, then rinse completely with warm water.

Moisturization: Keep your scalp hydrated by applying a lightweight conditioner or moisturizing treatment. Apply the conditioner to your hair's lengths and ends, avoiding the scalp to prevent accumulation. Use a leave-in conditioner or scalp serum containing nourishing elements to add more hydration.

Scalp Massage Techniques

Fingertip Massage: Use your fingertips to massage the scalp in circular strokes. Begin at the front hairline and work your way back to cover the entire scalp. Apply light to moderate pressure on the places where you feel tension or discomfort.

Kneading Motion: Using your thumb and fingers, knead tiny portions of the scalp gently in a circular motion. Apply mild pressure on the front, back, and sides of the head to improve circulation and relax the scalp muscles.

Tapping or Drumming: Gently tap or drum your fingertips against the scalp, switching hands. This approach stimulates blood flow and promotes relaxation.

Brush Massage: Using a scalp massage brush or a soft-bristled hairbrush, gently massage the scalp in circles. Begin at the front hairline and work your way back to cover the entire scalp. This procedure helps to exfoliate the scalp, distribute natural oils, and promote hair growth.

Frequency and Duration

When washing your hair, massage your scalp for at least 5 to 10 minutes. For best effects, incorporate scalp massage into your routine twice to three times each week.

Maintain a consistent scalp care and massage routine to encourage long-term hair growth and vitality.

Additional Tips:

To add nourishment and hydration to your scalp massage, use natural oils like coconut oil, jojoba oil, or argan oil.

Deep breathing or meditation while stroking your scalp will help you relax and lessen stress.

Excessive force or aggressive scratching of the scalp can cause skin irritation and hair follicle damage.

Be gentle with your hair and scalp, especially if you have sensitive skin or are experiencing hair loss. Listen to your body and modify the pressure and intensity of the massage as necessary.

Scalp care and massage techniques are vital components of a comprehensive strategy for supporting healthy hair development and scalp health. By implementing these methods into your normal hair care routine and tailoring them to your specific requirements, you may improve blood circulation, remove pollutants, and create an ideal environment for hair follicles to develop. Remember to be consistent, careful, and attentive to your scalp's needs to attain the finest long-term results.

Exercise and Physical Activity

Exercise and physical activity are not only necessary components of a healthy lifestyle, but they also play an important role in promoting hair health and reducing factors that contribute to hair loss. While exercise is not a direct cure for hair loss, it can help promote hair growth and scalp health through a variety of processes. In this complete overview, we'll look further into the relationship between exercise and hair health, including the advantages, types of workouts that are healthy, and practical tips for incorporating exercise into your daily routine.

Exercise enhances blood circulation all over the body, including the scalp. Increased blood flow to the scalp provides the oxygen, nutrients, and hormones required for healthy hair development. Adequate circulation also aids in the removal of toxins and waste products from the scalp, creating a clean and nourishing environment for hair follicles to thrive in.

Stress Reduction

Regular exercise is an effective stress reliever that can help lower levels of stress chemicals like cortisol. Chronic stress is a common cause of hair loss because it affects the hair development cycle, leading to disorders such as telogen effluvium and alopecia areata. Individuals who manage stress via exercise may be able to improve their hair health and create a healthier scalp environment.

Hormonal Balance.

Physical exercise can affect hormone levels in the body, which play an important role in hair development and maintenance. For example, regular exercise can help manage insulin levels, reduce insulin resistance, and balance hormone levels like testosterone and estrogen. Male and female pattern baldness are linked to hormonal abnormalities, including high amounts of dihydrotestosterone (DHT).

Enhanced Immune Function

Exercise helps to maintain a strong immune system, which is necessary for scalp health and the prevention of scalp infections and autoimmune illnesses like alopecia areata. A strong immune system helps protect hair follicles from injury and promotes healthy hair development.

Stimulation of Hair Follicle

Certain exercises, such as yoga and strength training, may indirectly stimulate hair follicles by increasing blood flow and massaging the scalp. Inversions and forward bends in yoga can increase circulation to the scalp, whereas scalp massage techniques integrated into strength training routines can encourage relaxation and scalp health.

Nutrient Delivery and Absorption

Exercise improves nutrient delivery and absorption throughout the body, including the scalp. A sufficient diet of important vitamins, minerals, and antioxidants is required for good hair development. Exercise can improve nutritional absorption by boosting digestion, metabolism, and cellular uptake, benefiting overall hair health.

Optimal hair growth conditions

Regular physical exercise promotes a healthy body weight and metabolism, which are critical for hormonal balance and overall health. Excess body weight and metabolic imbalances can lead to insulin resistance and inflammation, both of which can have a bad influence on hair health.

Walking, jogging, swimming, cycling, and dancing are all aerobic exercises that improve cardiovascular health and circulation throughout the body, including the scalp.

Strength Training: Resistance workouts with weights, resistance bands, or body weight serve to enhance muscle strength and improve metabolic health. Incorporating scalp massage techniques into strength training regimens can help to improve scalp health.

Yoga and Tai Chi are mind-body activities that use movement, breathing methods, and relaxation to relieve stress, increase flexibility, and improve general well-being. Certain yoga poses, such as downward dogs and headstands, can stimulate blood flow to the scalp and induce relaxation.

Incorporating Exercise in Your Routine

Aim for at least 150 minutes of moderate-intensity aerobic exercise or 75 minutes of vigorous-intensity aerobic exercise every week, according to health standards.

Choose things that you enjoy and can stick with over time to maintain consistency.

Incorporate scalp massage techniques or yoga positions that promote circulation and relaxation into your workout program to improve hair health.

Stay hydrated before, during, and after exercise to promote overall hydration and scalp health.

Exercise and physical activity are important components of a healthy lifestyle and can indirectly benefit hair health by boosting circulation, reducing stress, regulating hormones, and creating an optimal environment for hair growth. By incorporating regular exercise into your routine and selecting activities that encourage relaxation and circulation, you can improve scalp health and hair vitality. Furthermore, eating a well-balanced diet rich in important nutrients and using stress-management skills can enhance the benefits of exercise for general hair health.

CHAPTER FOUR

Incorporating Healthy Habits for Hair Growth

Practicing healthy habits is critical for supporting optimal hair development and preserving overall hair health. This comprehensive book delves into a variety of tactics, including sleep hygiene and its impact on hair development, avoiding dangerous behaviors, leveraging the benefits of essential oils and aromatherapy, and using home remedies. Consistency is essential while applying these strategies to get long-term outcomes. Individuals who follow these routines can help their hair grow faster and create a healthy scalp environment that promotes thick, colorful hair. Let's look deeper into each element to see how these behaviors can benefit hair health and growth.

Sleep Hygiene and Its Impact

Sleep hygiene encompasses the behaviors and habits that support healthy and restorative sleep. While many people prioritize nutrition and exercise for general health, the value of adequate sleep should not be overlooked.

Adequate sleep is essential for a variety of physiological activities, including cell regeneration, hormone control, and immunological response. In terms of hair health, adequate and restful sleep is critical in promoting the growth, strength, and vitality of hair follicles. In this comprehensive guide, we will look at the importance of sleep hygiene and how it affects hair health, as well as practical recommendations for improving sleep quality.

The Value of Sleep for Hair Health

Quality sleep allows the body to repair, renew, and revitalize cells, including those responsible for hair growth. The hair growth cycle is the process by which hair follicles grow, rest, and shed. During the restorative stages of sleep, such as deep sleep and REM (rapid eye movement), the body goes through several physiological processes that help hair follicles operate and promote healthy hair development.

Effects of Sleep Deprivation on Hair

Sleep deprivation or poor sleep quality can affect the body's normal functions, resulting in hormone imbalances, increased stress, and weakened immunity. These variables can contribute to several hair-related concerns, including:

Hair Thinning and Shedding: Lack of sleep can alter the hair growth cycle, resulting in greater shedding and lower hair density. Chronic sleep disruptions may contribute to conditions such as telogen effluvium, which occurs when hair enters the resting phase prematurely and is lost.

Inadequate sleep can inhibit hair growth because the body prioritizes critical tasks over non-essential ones, such as hair growth. This may result in shorter hair growth cycles and decreased total hair growth.

The effects of stress hormones.

Sleep deprivation can raise stress hormone levels, including cortisol, which can interrupt the hair development cycle and cause hair loss. Chronic stress and high cortisol levels can cause telogen effluvium, a condition in which hair follicles enter the resting phase early and lose more than usual.

Inflammation and Scalp Health.

Chronic sleep deprivation can cause systemic inflammation, compromising scalp health. Inflammation in the scalp can affect hair follicle activity, causing hair loss and scalp diseases such as dandruff and seborrheic dermatitis. Furthermore, inflammation can reduce blood circulation to the scalp, jeopardizing hair health.

Impact on Circulation

Quality sleep promotes healthy blood circulation, which delivers nutrients and oxygen to the scalp and hair follicles. Adequate blood flow is essential for preserving the health and vitality of hair follicles because it ensures nutrient delivery and waste disposal. Inadequate sleep can cause poor circulation, which deprives hair follicles of crucial nutrients, resulting in weakened hair and delayed development.

Promotion of Growth Hormones

Adequate sleep stimulates the release of growth hormones, particularly human growth hormone (HGH), which aids in tissue repair and regeneration, including hair follicle function. Optimal amounts of growth hormones promote healthy hair growth and maintenance.

Tips to Improve Sleep Hygiene

Improving sleep hygiene is developing habits and behaviors that encourage comfortable and refreshing sleep. Here are some tips to improve sleep quality:

Maintain a Consistent Sleep Schedule: To regulate your body's internal clock, go to bed and wake up at the same times every day, including weekends.

Create a soothing nighttime Routine: Set up a soothing nighttime routine to communicate to your body that it is time to unwind. This could include reading, having a warm bath, or using relaxation techniques such as deep breathing or meditation.

Create a Comfortable Sleep Environment: Keep your bedroom dark, quiet, and cool. Invest in a comfy mattress and pillows to promote healthy sleep.

Limit Screen Time Before Bed: Avoid using electronic gadgets like cellphones, computers, and televisions before bedtime since the blue light they emit interferes with melatonin production and disrupts sleep.

Avoid Stimulants Before Bed: Limit your intake of caffeine, nicotine, and alcohol close to bedtime, as these chemicals can impair sleep quality and disturb the sleep cycle.

Seeking Professional Help.

If you continue to have trouble sleeping despite applying healthy sleep hygiene measures, consult a healthcare practitioner. They can assist uncover underlying causes of sleep disorders and offer relevant actions or treatments.

Prioritizing proper sleep hygiene is critical for general health and promoting healthy hair development. Quality sleep boosts hormone balance, decreases stress, improves scalp health, and provides proper nutrient supply to hair follicles. Individuals can improve their hair health and overall well-being by developing appropriate sleep habits and dealing with sleep disruptions. Incorporating these habits into your routine can result in better sleep quality and healthier, more vivid hair over time.

Avoiding Harmful Habits

Avoiding hazardous practices is critical for the health and vitality of your hair. Certain activities and practices can hurt hair growth, resulting in thinning, breakage, and loss. In this detailed part, we'll look at typical dangerous habits to avoid and how they affect hair health:

Over styling and Heat Damage

Excessive use of styling products like flat irons, curling wands, and blow dryers can heat damage the hair cuticle, resulting in dryness, brittleness, and breaking. To avoid damage, avoid using high heat settings and limit the number of times you heat style.

Chemical Treatments

Chemical treatments such as perms, relaxers, and hair colors can damage the hair shaft and alter its natural structure. Overprocessing hair with strong chemicals can cause damage, breakage, and even hair loss. Consider using milder, more natural alternatives, or reducing the frequency of chemical treatments.

Tight Hairstyles and Hair Accessories.

Wearing hairstyles that pull on the hair, such as tight ponytails, braids, or buns, can put a strain on the hair follicles, resulting in traction alopecia. Similarly, employing too-tight hair accessories such as elastic bands or clips can cause breakage and damage. To reduce hair strain, opt for looser hairstyles and mild hair accessories.

Poor Nutrition.

A diet low in critical nutrients can harm hair health and contribute to problems like thinning and dullness. Avoiding dangerous dietary habits including overconsumption of processed meals, sugary snacks, and bad fats will assist promote healthy hair growth. Instead, focus on eating a well-balanced diet high in vitamins, minerals, and protein to nourish your hair from the inside.

Smoking and excessive alcohol consumption

Smoking and excessive alcohol use can hurt overall health, including hair health. Smoking reduces blood flow to the scalp, depriving hair follicles of vital nutrients and oxygen. Similarly, excessive alcohol intake can cause dehydration, vitamin deficiencies, and hormonal abnormalities, all of which hurt hair development.

Stress & Anxiety

Chronic stress and worry can cause hormonal imbalances and alter the hair development cycle, resulting in more shedding and hair loss. Finding healthy ways to manage stress, such as practicing relaxation techniques, exercising, or seeking help from a therapist, can help to reduce its impact on hair health.

Skipping Regular Hair Care

Neglecting routine hair care techniques like shampooing, conditioning, and moisturizing can cause a buildup of oil, grime, and product residue on the scalp and hair, clogging pores and impeding hair development. Establishing a consistent hair care routine that is specific to your hair type and needs is critical for preserving scalp health and fostering optimal hair development.

Sleep deprivation

Inadequate sleep can disturb hormone balance, raise stress, and damage general health, all of which have a detrimental impact on hair growth. Prioritizing quality sleep and maintaining good sleep hygiene habits can promote healthy hair growth and general well-being.

Avoiding hazardous practices is critical for the health and vitality of your hair. By being aware of frequent harmful behaviors and making intentional steps to avoid them, you can encourage healthy hair growth, strength, and resistance. Healthy habits like gentle styling, a balanced diet, stress management strategies, and consistent hair care routines can all contribute to long-term hair health and vitality.

Essential Oils and Aromatherapy

Essential oils contain a variety of ingredients that are known to enhance and maintain hair health. They also offer natural remedies for many common hair problems and may be favored by individuals who want to avoid potentially dangerous chemicals or synthetics in hair care.

Certain essential oils have been shown to improve scalp and hair cleanliness, brightness, and growth, but these effects are thought to occur in a variety of ways. The therapeutic effects of these oils can be linked to their primary ingredients and their synergistic interactions.

When using essential oils in hair care, it is important to analyze the qualities of each oil to determine how they can best address particular hair requirements and goals.

Atlas Cedarwood, Carrot Seed, Ylang Ylang, Clary Sage, Rosemary, and Tea Tree are some of the most commonly utilized essential oils in hair care products and routines. Each of these oils has distinct chemical profiles that indicate its recommended usage for hair; for example, Rosemary Oil is renowned for renewing all hair types, Carrot Seed Oil is recognized for its hair protection properties, and Ylang Ylang Oil is known for balancing both dry and oily hair.

Nourishing Hair Care Benefits of Essential Oils

Many of us strive to have soft, shiny, and healthy hair. Hair is regarded to be an important indicator of one's internal health, and it can also have a big impact on one's attractiveness, confidence, and overall demeanor. Even though our hair serves an important protective function by keeping us warm and providing a barrier against external pollutants or injury, the hair strands and scalp require adequate protection from factors such as harsh styling, inclement weather, excessive washing, and aggressive cosmetic ingredients. Dryness, dullness, damage, split ends, and hair loss are all caused in part by the harmful impacts of these external components.

Essential oils have long been utilized in both traditional and mainstream hair care to improve hair quality and cosmetic appeal. These oils' diverse compositions, combined with their consequent qualities, can naturally cleanse, hydrate, soothe, balance, bring out the vibrancy of hair color, and perform a variety of other beneficial hair care tasks. Many commercial hair care brands employ essential oils because of their natural benefits. Herbalists employ essential oils in holistic medicines to treat alopecia, hair breakage, and even premature graying.

Regardless of hair type, condition, or personal hair objectives, these all-natural volatile oils can be extremely nourishing and even reparative for an improved feel and appearance, as well as healthy hair development!

How Essential Oils Help Your Hair

Essential oils can improve the appearance and health of our hair in a variety of ways. They can primarily contribute by:

1. Supporting the cleansing and detoxification of the scalp and hair strands
2. Increasing hair growth using rubefacient or stimulatory properties (e.g., Rosemary Oil)
3. Soothing scalp irritations, itching, and scabbing
4. Adding gloss and healthy luster to strands
5. Balance the natural hair oils to enhance the appearance of brittle or oily hair.
6. Chamomile oil brightens blond hair, while rosemary and sage oil enhance darker hair tones.
7. Helping to treat, moisturize, detangle, or style hair
8. Calming the emotions or senses, thereby indirectly increasing hair health via stress reduction.

As can be seen, essential oils have a wide range of applications. In addition to these benefits, essential oils are popular in hair care and cosmetics because they scent the hair with appealing aromas while eliminating the need for synthetic fragrances. Many people love including these oils into their hair treatments because of their fragrant properties, which can stimulate emotions of self-care and mental refreshment.

ATLAS CEDARWOOD ESSENTIAL OIL - Naturally reduces dandruff and hair loss.

This essential oil, distilled from fragrant Atlas Cedarwood (Cedrus atlantica), has a strengthening quality and has been shown to help with dandruff, hair loss, and irritated scalps. Cedarwood Oil cleanses and relaxes the scalp, allowing it to release or rebalance its natural oils, resulting in smoother, softer, and shinier hair. Its mild purifying characteristics aid in hair washing and a few drops can be added to a single shampoo application for naturally clean and revitalized locks.

Chemically, Atlas Cedarwood Oil is high in sesquiterpenes, particularly Himachalenes, which are thought to have circulatory effects. These elements are thought to stimulate the follicles and aid in hair loss. Indeed, this woodsy oil has shown promise in slowing hair loss in people with alopecia areata, a disease that causes patchy areas of fall-out. This improvement was observed in some people who had a daily scalp massage with a stimulating blend of Cedarwood, Thyme, Rosemary, and Lavender oils. Cedarwood's fresh, sweet, earthy, unisex smell appeals to both men and women looking to include a naturally nourishing hair regimen.

CARROT SEED ESSENTIAL OIL - Invigorates and rejuvenates oily or damaged hair.

Carrot Seed Oil is derived from the dried seeds of Daucus carota, an ethereal-looking plant with white blossoms that is also known as 'Wild Carrot' or 'Bishop's Lace'. This musky, earthy essential oil is particularly protective due to its antioxidant and regenerative properties, thus it is frequently recommended for persons with aged skin. Hair that has suffered from free radical damage, resulting in rough, dull, thinning strands, will benefit from Carrot Seed

Oil's nourishing characteristics, especially when combined with leave-on treatments such as hair masks, serums, or conditioners.

This oil's active components include Alpha-Pinene and Carotol. Alpha-pinene, a monoterpene, is known for its cleaning, anti-inflammatory, and antioxidant properties. This component also aids in oil regulation and can be a beneficial oil for persons with greasy scalps. Carotol, another key ingredient in this oil, is a sesquiterpenoid molecule best recognized for its antifungal properties. It can help those with scalp yeast and fungal diseases, such as dandruff.

CLARY SAGE ESSENTIAL OIL - Naturally promotes hair growth and clarifies oily hair.

Clary Sage Oil, also known as a valuable 'Woman's Oil,' has numerous medicinal properties that can benefit one's general health and beauty. This harmonizing essential oil has a restorative and balancing effect and is said to reduce sebum, soothe irritated scalps, and gently stimulate new hair growth. Clary Sage Oil is widely promoted as a natural cure for female hair loss due to its putative effects on the endocrine system, which are frequently linked to one of its ingredients, Sclareol. Imbalances in certain hormones, such as estrogen, can cause issues with hair growth, thinning, or shedding. However, there could be a more psychosomatic rationale for these claims; Clary Sage Oil's floral, sweet, and earthy aroma can be deeply calming and uplifting, thereby reducing the harmful effects of stress on hair development. As a result, this oil contains a high concentration of Linalyl Acetate and Linalool, which have been shown to work together to produce psychologically relaxing and calming effects.

YLANG YLANG ESSENTIAL OIL - Balances both oily and dry hair types.

Ylang Ylang Oil, distilled from the curly yellow blossoms of the tropical Cananga odorata, is known for its powerful balancing properties and is said to have a harmonizing impact on both the skin and hair surfaces. In the Victorian era, Ylang Ylang Oil was combined with coconut or palm oil to create the legendary Macassar hair oil, which was used for conditioning and style, notably by Victorian males.

Intriguingly, because of its balancing effects, Ylang Ylang Oil is advised for both oily and acne-prone skin types, as well as those with excessively dry skin - a recommendation that also applies to hair kinds. This lovely flower oil is suitable for oily, dry, and normal hair types. It not only perfumes the strands with its exotic, sensual aroma, but it also helps regulate sebum levels, functioning as a natural hair tonic that promotes shine, volume, and general manageability.

It's worth noting that Ylang Ylang Oil is extracted using a complex fractional distillation process, with Ylang Ylang Extra being the first distillate produced. Subsequent distillates are referred to as Ylang Ylang 1, 2, and 3, respectively; these types differ in terms of scent intensity (Ylang Ylang 1 being the most intense) and chemical composition. Ylang Ylang 1 contains a larger concentration of Linalool and esters, such as Geranyl acetate, which are anti-inflammatory and pain-relieving, making it useful for relaxing hair care. On the other hand, Ylang Ylang 3 is high in sesquiterpenes, which are known to improve circulation and have purifying characteristics, making it effective in a variety of hair applications ranging from cleansing to hair development.

ROSEMARY ESSENTIAL OIL - Naturally promotes hair growth and rejuvenates all hair types.

The botanical extract and volatile oil of the Rosemary plant are among the most commonly used natural components in hair products. This vivid oil has an exhilarating spicy-herbal scent and is extremely stimulating in its properties. Its widespread use is due to its potent stimulatory properties on both the skin and the hair, which increase blood circulation and encourage hair growth. Furthermore, Rosemary Oil cleanses and calms the scalp, removing dandruff, grime, sweat, and buildup. This treasured oil is also known to provide shine, depth, and luster to the hair, especially for individuals with darker hair. It is also regarded as a must-have essential oil for people with long hair due to its strengthening characteristics, which help prevent hair breakage and split ends.

Rosemary Oil contains a high concentration of oxides, monoterpenes, and ketones, such as 1,8-cineole, Alpha-Pinene, and camphor. These ingredients give essential oil cleaning, anti-inflammatory, circulation-boosting, and lice-repellent characteristics, making it an extremely important ingredient in almost all hair care regimens.

TEA TREE ESSENTIAL OIL - Balances Scalp, Cleans Hair, & Eliminates Lice

Derived from the leaves of the Tea Tree plant (Melaleuca alternifolia), this essential oil has a strong reputation as a natural antibacterial, making it very good for scalp health. Its inherent antibacterial and antifungal properties may be therapeutic, particularly for those suffering from dandruff and scalp infections. Its anti-seborrheic characteristics assist in soothing the scalp by reducing flakiness, scaliness, and soreness. Tea Tree Oil has also been traditionally used to treat hair lice; 2-3 drops of this essential oil mixed with suitable carrier oil and gently combed through to disperse throughout the scalp and strands is thought to kill lice if done daily for many days.

Tea Tree Oil's ability to clear scalp debris contributes to its hair growth benefits. Sweat, skin cells, styling products, dirt, and other residues can clog hair follicles, slowing hair growth. Tea Tree Oil's strong purifying and clarifying properties help cleanse the scalp and unclog follicles, allowing for more hair growth and length.

Tea Tree Oil is another oil that works well for both dry and oily hair. Its anti-inflammatory and relaxing properties might help those with dry hair and scalps avoid irritations and itching. Its cleaning properties assist those with greasy hair in removing extra sebum.

Lavender Oil: In addition to its calming aroma, lavender oil offers antibacterial characteristics that can aid in the maintenance of a healthy scalp and the promotion of hair development.

Peppermint Oil: Peppermint oil cools the scalp and may promote circulation. It is often used to soothe scalp inflammation, promote hair growth, and offer a fresh aroma to hair care products.

Lemongrass Essential Oil

Dandruff is a frequent illness, and having a healthy, flake-free scalp is essential for hair health. Lemongrass oil is an excellent dandruff treatment, with one 2015 study showing that it decreased dandruff considerably after one week.

Lemongrass oil for dandruff works best when applied every day. Every day, add a few drops to your shampoo or conditioner and massage them into your scalp.

Thyme Essential Oil

Thyme can stimulate the scalp while also actively preventing hair loss, hence promoting hair growth. Thyme oil, like cedarwood oil, has been shown to help treat alopecia areata.Trusted source.

Thyme is especially potent, even among essential oils. Before applying to your scalp, mix only two little drops with two tablespoons of carrier oil. Leave it on for around 10 minutes before washing it away.

DIY Recipes for Hair Growth Blend with essential and carrier oils.

Essential oil hair oil mixtures are said to contain therapeutic characteristics that might boost hair and scalp health. However, it is critical to utilize them responsibly and conduct a patch test before applying them to your scalp. Here are some essential oil recipes that promote hair growth:

Recipe 1: Nourishing Hair-Growth Blend.

Ingredients:

Two tablespoons of fractionated coconut oil.

Five drops of Rosemary essential oil

Five drops of Geranium essential oil.

Three drops of Cedarwood essential oil.

Instructions:

In a small glass bottle, combine the Jojoba oil with the Rosemary, Lavender, and Cedarwood essential oils.

Mix lightly to ensure that all of the oils are incorporated.

Apply a few drops of this combination to your scalp and massage it gently in circular strokes. This increases blood flow and benefits hair.

Apply the combination to your scalp for at least 30 minutes. It is best to leave it overnight for optimal absorption.

Rinse your hair completely with a mild shampoo and conditioner to remove any oil residue, resulting in smoother and shinier hair.

Before using the blend, perform a tiny patch test on your forearm to ensure there are no adverse reactions. This is advised because the combination contains numerous components.

Recipe 2: Strengthening and Stimulating Scalp Massage Oil.

Ingredients:

Five drops of peppermint essential oil.

5 drops of Eucalyptus essential oil.

3 drops of Tea Tree Essential Oil

Two tablespoons of jojoba oil.

Instructions:

Place the recommended amount of jojoba oil in a basin.

Combine it with peppermint, eucalyptus, and tea tree essential oils.

Combine the oils to ensure homogeneity.

Apply the oil mixture immediately to the scalp. It can be applied from root to tip.

Gently massage your scalp for 5 to 10 minutes to increase blood circulation.

If you apply the oil to your scalp in the morning, leave it on for at least 30 minutes. Wash it off with a gentle shampoo. The special blend may prevent hair breakage and result in thicker-looking hair.

Before using the blend, perform a tiny patch test on your forearm to ensure there are no adverse reactions. This is advised because the combination contains numerous components.

Recipe 3: Revitalizing Hair Growth Spray.

Ingredients:

10 drops of eucalyptus essential oil.

10 drops of Roman Chamomile Essential Oil

1/2 cup distilled water.

Use 1 tablespoon of Aloe Vera Gel.

Grab a spray bottle or spritzer. Combine the ingredients: distilled water, aloe vera gel, eucalyptus oil, and Roman chamomile essential oil.

Close the bottle and shake vigorously to ensure that all of the components are combined. Remember, it contains Aloe Vera, so shake it well.

First, establish a regular hair care routine that includes shampooing and conditioning your hair. Next, use a towel to dry the hair, leaving it somewhat damp.

Spritz the mixture onto your scalp.

Massage for several minutes to increase blood flow and absorption. These natural oils can help promote a healthy scalp.

This time, let your hair air dry. It is best to avoid using heat-styling tools just after the application.

Before using the blend, perform a tiny patch test on your forearm to ensure there are no adverse reactions. This is advised because the combination contains numerous components.

Recipe 4: Hair Growth Hot Oil Treatment.

Ingredients:

four drops of eucalyptus essential oil

Four drops of frankincense essential oil.

2 tablespoons of coconut oil.

2 tablespoons of castor oil.

Instructions:

Create a makeshift double boiler by inserting a small heat-safe bowl into a bigger dish filled with hot water.

In a smaller bowl, blend the coconut and castor oils.

Heat the oils until they are somewhat warm, but not hot enough to burn the skin.

Next, combine the Peppermint and Rosemary essential oils with the heated oil.

Stir carefully to ensure that all of the oils are thoroughly combined.

Apply the heated oil mixture to the scalp and hair. Make sure it reaches the corners.

Massage your scalp gently for 5 to 10 minutes. This promotes blood circulation and improves absorption. The ricinoleic acid in castor oil dilates blood arteries, improving blood flow.

Wrap your hair in a warm towel after applying oil to the entire scalp and hair.

Leave it on for at least 30 to 60 minutes.

To eliminate the oil from your hair, shampoo and condition it as usual.

Before using the blend, perform a tiny patch test on your forearm to ensure there are no adverse reactions. This is advised because the combination contains numerous components.

Recipe 5: Revitalizing Hair Growth Blend Serum.

Ingredients:

Two tablespoons of argan oil.

Five drops of Clary Sage essential oil.

Five drops of Cedarwood essential oil.

Three drops of Thyme essential oil.

Instructions:

Combine all of the oils and store them in a dark-colored glass.

Close the bottle and shake vigorously to completely combine the oils. Do this before each use.

Apply the heated oil mixture to the scalp and hair. Make sure it reaches the roots.

For several minutes, gently massage the serum into your scalp with your fingertips. Use a scalp massager to increase the reach and stimulation of hair follicles.

Leave it on for at least 30 to 60 minutes. For the greatest results, leave it overnight.

The next day (or after half an hour), wash your hair with a gentle shampoo and conditioner to remove any oil residue.

Before using the blend, perform a tiny patch test on your forearm to ensure there are no adverse reactions. This is advised because the combination contains numerous components.

Aromatherapy for Hair care

Scalp Massage: Mixing a few drops of essential oil with carrier oil (such as coconut or jojoba oil) and rubbing it into the scalp will assist increase circulation, nourishing the hair follicles, and promoting relaxation. Scalp massage with aromatherapy oils can be added to your normal hair care regimen for additional advantages.

Hair Rinse: Diluting essential oils in water and applying the mixture as a hair rinse after shampooing can offer a nice aroma to the hair while also benefiting the scalp and hair health. Certain essential oils, such as rosemary and lavender, are very useful for this purpose.

Hair Masks: Adding essential oils to homemade hair masks or commercial hair care products can boost their nourishing and rejuvenating effects. For example, combining a few drops of rosemary oil with a natural hair conditioner can help to strengthen the hair and improve its overall appearance.

Application Tip:

Essential oils are highly concentrated and strong, thus they must be adequately diluted before application to the skin or scalp. Mix essential oils with carrier oil, water, or hair care products at the suggested dilution ratios.

Patch Test: Before using any essential oil on your scalp or hair, test a tiny area of skin for any bad reactions or sensitivities.

Avoid Contact with Eyes: Keep essential oils away from your eyes because they can irritate them. If contact is made, thoroughly rinse with water.

Consultation: Before using essential oils for hair care, check with your doctor if you have any underlying health conditions, pregnant, or breastfeeding.

Home remedies provide natural and easily accessible methods for improving scalp health, nourishing hair follicles, and increasing hair growth. These cures frequently use ordinary kitchen or garden products, making them easy and inexpensive ways to keep your hair healthy. Let's look at some popular home remedies and their benefits for hair care.

Coconut Oil.

Benefits: Coconut oil contains fatty acids that permeate the hair shaft, providing hydration and nourishment. It moisturizes dry hair, reduces protein loss, and promotes overall hair health.

Application: Warm coconut oil and apply it to your scalp and hair as a pre-shampoo therapy. Leave it on for at least 30 minutes or overnight for best results, then shampoo and condition as usual.

Aloe Vera.

Benefits: Aloe vera gel includes enzymes that improve scalp health by eliminating dead skin cells and decreasing inflammation. It relaxes the scalp, hydrates dry hair, and promotes hair development.

Application: Gently massage fresh aloe vera gel into the scalp and hair. Leave it on for 30 to 60 minutes, then rinse with lukewarm water. To achieve the best effects, repeat 2-3 times per week.

Rinse with apple cider vinegar (ACV).

Benefits: ACV balances the pH of the scalp, removes buildup, and clarifies hair. It restores luster, minimizes frizz, and promotes scalp health.

Application: Combine equal parts ACV and water and use as a final rinse after shampooing. Let it stay for a few minutes before rinsing with water. Use once or twice a week to keep the scalp healthy.

Onion Juice.

Benefits: Onion juice includes sulfur components that stimulate hair follicles and encourage growth. It strengthens hair, lowers hair loss, and increases overall density.

Application: Extract the onion juice and apply it directly to the scalp with a cotton pad or applicator. Leave it on for 15-30 minutes, then shampoo and condition normally. To achieve the best effects, use 2-3 times weekly.

Egg mask

Benefits: Eggs include protein, vitamins, and minerals, which nourish and encourage hair development. An egg mask fortifies hair, adds gloss, and enhances texture.

Application: Make a hair mask by beating an egg and mixing it with olive oil or honey. Apply the mixture to moist hair, concentrating on the scalp and the roots. Leave it on for 30 to 60 minutes, then rinse with cold water and shampoo.

Importance of Consistency

Consistency is essential for attaining the desired outcomes with home remedies for hair care. While these cures provide natural and efficient answers, they frequently produce slow benefits that necessitate continued application over time. Here's why consistency is important for healthy hair:

Gradual results.

Home treatments produce modest results, and consistent use is required to observe major improvements in hair health. You may increase the effectiveness of these cures by including them in your daily hair care routine and following them consistently.

Maintaining Scalp Health.

Consistency is vital for maintaining scalp health and treating typical scalp problems like dryness, dandruff, and inflammation. Regular use of home treatments can assist in maintaining the scalp hydrated, balanced, and free of buildup.

Promoting Hair Growth.

Many home remedies stimulate hair follicles, increase circulation to the scalp, and encourage hair growth. Consistently employing these solutions may result in thicker, fuller hair over time by feeding the scalp and promoting healthy hair growth.

Preventing Damage

Consistent use of natural components can help prevent damage to the hair and scalp caused by environmental factors, heat style, or chemical treatments. By using gentle, nourishing therapies, you may keep your hair in good condition and reduce breakage and split ends.

Tips For Consistency.

To maintain consistency in your hair care practice and maximize the benefits of home remedies, consider the following tips:

Establish a routine.

Incorporate home remedies into your normal hair care routine by setting aside specified days or times for treatment. Consistency is easier to maintain when treatments become a regular component of your grooming routine.

Keep the ingredients accessible.

Stock up on essential ingredients for your favorite home cures so that you always have them on hand when needed.

Having components easily available makes it easier to stick to your hair care regimen.

Track your progress.

Keep track of your hair's progress by taking photos or writing down any changes you see over time. Monitoring changes in hair texture, growth, and overall health can help keep you motivated and committed to your hair care routine.

Be patient.

Consistency is essential, but results may not appear overnight. Be patient and allow your hair time to respond to the treatments. With constant application, you should see a gradual improvement in hair health and growth.

Home remedies are natural and efficient ways to promote scalp and hair health. Consistency in applying these remedies is vital for attaining the intended outcomes, whether it's strengthening the hair, stimulating growth, or improving general hair health. By introducing home remedies into your normal hair care routine and following to them consistently, you can gradually cultivate healthier, stronger hair over time.

Conclusion

Natural therapies are a potential option for anyone looking to cure hair loss and encourage thicker, more resilient hair. Throughout this book, we've looked at a variety of options, including herbal remedies, scalp care techniques, stress management measures, essential oils, and home remedies, each with its own set of benefits for addressing the root reasons for hair loss and promoting regrowth.

Understanding the many types and reasons for hair loss allows people to adjust their strategy to include natural therapies that target particular elements contributing to their hair loss. Natural therapies offer holistic solutions that nourish hair from the inside out, whether they address hormonal imbalances, improve scalp health, stimulate circulation, or reduce stress.

Consistency appears as an important aspect of the effectiveness of natural hair loss treatments. A good hair care routine requires regular treatment application, attention to healthy lifestyle practices, and patience while viewing results. While natural therapies do not provide instant results, their mild and nourishing features can lead to considerable changes in hair health over time when used regularly.

Furthermore, using natural therapies for hair loss has advantages beyond regeneration. These solutions frequently boost general scalp health, improve hair texture and shine, and reduce the danger of negative side effects caused by harsh chemicals found in traditional hair care products.

It is critical to approach natural remedies with realistic expectations and to check with healthcare specialists or dermatologists, particularly in cases of severe or recurrent hair loss. Furthermore, combining natural therapies with a holistic approach to well-being, such as a healthy diet, regular exercise, stress management skills, and enough sleep, can boost their effectiveness in reversing hair loss and increasing overall well-being.

Natural therapies offer a mild yet effective way to reverse hair loss and promote healthier, more colorful hair. Individuals who incorporate these remedies into a thorough hair care regimen and apply them consistently can embark on a transforming journey toward restoring confidence in their hair and attaining long-term outcomes in their pursuit of optimal hair health.